Contents

Updated Estimates of the Effects of the Insurance Coverage Provisions of the Affordable Care Act, April 2014

Summary

The Congressional Budget Office (CBO) and the staff of the Joint Committee on Taxation (JCT) have updated their estimates of the budgetary effects of the provisions of the Affordable Care Act (ACA) that relate to health insurance coverage. The new estimates, which are included in CBO's latest baseline projections, reflect CBO's most recent economic forecast, account for administrative actions taken and regulations issued through March 2014, and incorporate new data and various modeling updates.[1]

Relative to their previous projections, CBO and JCT now estimate that the ACA's coverage provisions will result in lower net costs to the federal government: The agencies now project a net cost of $36 billion for 2014, $5 billion less than the previous projection for the year; and $1,383 billion for the 2015–2024 period, $104 billion less than the previous projection.[2]

The estimated net costs for 2014 stem almost entirely from spending for subsidies that are to be provided through insurance exchanges (often called marketplaces) and from an increase in spending for Medicaid (see Table 1). For the 2015–2024 period, the projected net costs consist of the following:

■ Gross costs of $1,839 billion for subsidies and related spending for insurance obtained through the exchanges, Medicaid, the Children's Health Insurance Program (CHIP), and tax credits for small employers; and

■ A partial offset of $456 billion in receipts from penalty payments, additional revenues resulting from the excise tax on high-premium insurance plans, and the effects on income and payroll tax revenues and associated outlays arising from projected changes in employer coverage.

Those estimates address only the insurance coverage provisions of the ACA, which do not generate all of the act's budgetary effects. Many other provisions, on net, are expected to reduce budget deficits. Considering all of the provisions—including the coverage provisions—CBO and JCT estimated in July 2012 (their most recent comprehensive estimate) that the ACA's overall effect would be to reduce federal deficits.[3]

---

1. For CBO's latest baseline projections, see Congressional Budget Office, *Updated Budget Projections: 2014 to 2024* (April 2014), www.cbo.gov/publication/45229.

2. For CBO and JCT's previous projections of the effects of the ACA's insurance coverage provisions, see Congressional Budget Office, *The Budget and Economic Outlook: 2014 to 2024*, Appendix B (February 2014), www.cbo.gov/publication/45010.

3. See Congressional Budget Office, letter to the Honorable John Boehner providing an estimate for H.R. 6079, the Repeal of Obamacare Act (July 24, 2012), www.cbo.gov/publication/43471. CBO and JCT can no longer determine exactly how the provisions of the ACA that are not related to the expansion of health insurance coverage have affected their projections of direct spending and revenues. The provisions that expand insurance coverage established entirely new programs or components of programs that can be isolated and reassessed. In contrast, other provisions of the ACA significantly modified existing federal programs and made changes to the Internal Revenue Code. Isolating the incremental effects of those provisions on previously existing programs and revenues four years after enactment of the ACA is not possible.

Table 1.

Effects on the Deficit of the Insurance Coverage Provisions of the Affordable Care Act

(Billions of dollars, by fiscal year)

	2014	2015	2016	2017	2018	2019	2020	2021	2022	2023	2024	Total, 2015– 2024
Exchange Subsidies and Related Spending[a]	17	36	77	94	101	107	112	119	125	129	132	1,032
Medicaid and CHIP Outlays[b]	20	42	62	70	77	82	84	87	91	96	101	792
Small-Employer Tax Credits[c]	1	2	1	1	1	1	1	2	2	2	2	15
Gross Cost of Coverage Provisions	38	80	141	164	180	190	197	208	218	227	235	1,839
Penalty Payments by Uninsured People	*	-2	-4	-4	-4	-5	-5	-5	-5	-6	-6	-46
Penalty Payments by Employers[c]	0	0	-8	-12	-13	-15	-16	-17	-18	-20	-21	-139
Excise Tax on High-Premium Insurance Plans[c]	0	0	0	0	-5	-10	-13	-16	-20	-25	-30	-120
Other Effects on Revenues and Outlays[d]	-2	-3	-6	-11	-14	-16	-18	-20	-21	-21	-22	-152
Net Cost of Coverage Provisions	**36**	**74**	**123**	**138**	**143**	**144**	**146**	**150**	**153**	**155**	**156**	**1,383**
Memorandum:												
Changes in Mandatory Spending	35	92	147	173	181	192	200	211	221	230	238	1,885
Changes in Revenues[e]	-1	18	24	35	37	48	54	61	68	75	83	503

Sources: Congressional Budget Office; staff of the Joint Committee on Taxation.

Notes: These numbers exclude effects on the deficit of provisions of the Affordable Care Act that are not related to insurance coverage. They also exclude federal administrative costs subject to appropriation. (CBO has previously estimated that the Internal Revenue Service would need to spend between $5 billion and $10 billion over the 2010–2019 period to implement the Affordable Care Act and that the Department of Health and Human Services and other federal agencies would also need to spend $5 billion to $10 billion over that period.) In addition, the Affordable Care Act included explicit authorizations for spending on a variety of grant and other programs; that funding is also subject to future appropriation action.

Unless otherwise noted, positive numbers indicate an increase in the deficit, and negative numbers indicate a decrease in the deficit.

CHIP = Children's Health Insurance Program; * = between zero and -$500 million.

a. Includes spending for exchange grants to states and net collections and payments for risk adjustment, reinsurance, and risk corridors.

b. Under current law, states have the flexibility to make programmatic and other budgetary changes to Medicaid and CHIP. CBO estimates that state spending on Medicaid and CHIP over the 2015–2024 period will be about $46 billion higher because of the coverage provisions of the Affordable Care Act than it would be otherwise.

c. These effects on the deficit include the associated effects of changes in taxable compensation on revenues.

d. Consists mainly of the effects of changes in taxable compensation on revenues. CBO estimates that outlays for Social Security benefits will increase by about $7 billion over the 2015–2024 period and that the coverage provisions will have negligible effects on outlays for other federal programs.

e. Positive numbers indicate an increase in revenues, and negative numbers indicate a decrease in revenues.

CBO and JCT have updated their baseline estimates of the budgetary effects of the ACA's insurance coverage provisions many times since that legislation was enacted in March 2010. As time has passed, the period spanned by the estimates has changed. But a year-by-year comparison shows that CBO and JCT's estimates of the net budgetary impact of the ACA's insurance coverage provisions have decreased, on balance, over the past four years.

This report describes the insurance coverage provisions of the ACA and CBO and JCT's current estimates of the budgetary effects of those provisions. That discussion is followed by an explanation of how and why those estimates differ from the interim estimates in CBO's February 2014 baseline. The report concludes with a discussion of the ways in which current estimates of the ACA's coverage provisions differ from those made when the law was enacted in March 2010.

The Insurance Coverage Provisions and Their Effects on the Number of People With and Without Insurance

Among the key elements of the ACA's insurance coverage provisions that are encompassed by the estimates discussed here are the following:

■ The ACA allows many individuals and families to purchase subsidized insurance through the exchanges (or marketplaces) operated either by the federal government or by a state government.

■ States are permitted but not required to expand eligibility for Medicaid.

■ Most legal residents of the United States must either obtain health insurance or pay a penalty for not doing so (under a provision known as the individual mandate).

■ Certain employers that decline to offer their employees health insurance coverage that meets specified standards will be assessed penalties.

■ A federal excise tax will be imposed on some health insurance plans with high premiums.

■ Most insurers offering policies either for purchase through the exchanges or directly to consumers outside of the exchanges must meet several requirements: For example, they must accept all applicants regardless of health status; they may vary premiums only by age, smoking status, and geographic location; and they may not limit coverage for preexisting medical conditions.[4]

■ Certain small employers that provide health insurance to their employees will be eligible to receive a tax credit of up to 50 percent of the cost of that insurance.

The ACA also made other changes to rules governing health insurance coverage that are not listed here. Those other provisions address coverage in the nongroup, small-group, and large-group markets, in some cases including self-insured employment-based plans.

CBO and JCT estimate that the insurance coverage provisions of the ACA will increase the proportion of the nonelderly population with insurance from roughly 80 percent in the absence of the ACA to about 84 percent in 2014 and to about 89 percent in 2016 and beyond (see Table 2). CBO and JCT project that 12 million more nonelderly people will have health insurance in 2014 than would have had it in the absence of the ACA. They also project that 19 million more people will be insured in 2015, 25 million more will be insured in 2016, and 26 million more will be insured each year from 2017 through 2024 than would have been the case without the ACA.

Those gains in coverage will be the net result of many changes in insurance coverage relative to what would have occurred in the absence of the ACA. In 2018 and later years, 25 million people are projected to have coverage through the exchanges, and 13 million more, on net, are projected to have coverage through Medicaid and CHIP than would have had it in the absence of the ACA. Partly offsetting those increases, however, are projected net decreases in employment-based coverage and in coverage in the nongroup market outside the exchanges.

The estimated increase in insurance coverage in 2014 represents the number of people who are expected to be insured this year under current law minus the number who would have been insured this year in the absence of the ACA. That number may differ from the number of people who are expected to be insured this year minus the number who were insured last year, because people move in and out of insurance coverage over time as a result of changes in employment, family circumstances, and other factors. In particular, some people who had insurance coverage in 2013 and would have become uninsured in 2014 for one reason or another in the absence of the ACA will, under the ACA, be covered in 2014 through the exchanges, Medicaid, or CHIP. Those people are included in CBO and JCT's estimate of the increase in insurance coverage in 2014 that stems from the ACA.[5] CBO and JCT have not estimated the number of people who were uninsured in 2013 and will be insured in 2014.

---

4. Premiums charged for adults 21 or older may not vary according to age by a ratio of more than 3:1.

5. Correspondingly, people who were uninsured in 2013 but would have obtained insurance in 2014 in the absence of the ACA are not counted as part of the increase in insurance coverage resulting from the ACA.

Table 2.

Effects of the Affordable Care Act on Health Insurance Coverage

(Millions of nonelderly people, by calendar year)

	2014	2015	2016	2017	2018	2019	2020	2021	2022	2023	2024
Insurance Coverage Without the ACA[a]											
Medicaid and CHIP	35	35	34	33	33	34	34	34	35	35	35
Employment-based coverage	156	158	160	163	164	165	165	165	166	166	166
Nongroup and other coverage[b]	24	24	25	25	26	26	26	26	27	27	27
Uninsured[c]	54	55	55	55	55	56	56	56	57	57	57
Total	270	272	274	277	278	280	281	282	283	284	285
Change in Insurance Coverage Under the ACA											
Insurance exchanges	6	13	24	25	25	25	25	25	25	25	25
Medicaid and CHIP	7	11	12	12	13	13	13	13	13	13	13
Employment-based coverage[d]	*	-2	-7	-7	-8	-8	-8	-8	-8	-7	-7
Nongroup and other coverage[b]	-1	-3	-4	-4	-4	-4	-4	-4	-4	-5	-5
Uninsured[c]	-12	-19	-25	-26	-26	-26	-26	-26	-26	-26	-26
Uninsured Under the ACA											
Number of uninsured nonelderly people[c]	42	36	30	30	29	30	30	30	31	31	31
Insured as a percentage of the nonelderly population											
Including all U.S. residents	84	87	89	89	89	89	89	89	89	89	89
Excluding unauthorized immigrants	86	89	91	92	92	92	92	92	92	92	92
Memorandum:											
Exchange Enrollees and Subsidies											
Number with unaffordable offer from employer[e]	**	**	**	**	**	**	**	**	**	**	**
Number of unsubsidized exchange enrollees (Millions of people)[f]	1	3	5	6	6	6	6	6	6	6	6
Average exchange subsidy per subsidized enrollee (Dollars)	4,410	4,250	4,830	4,930	5,300	5,570	5,880	6,220	6,580	6,890	7,170

Sources: Congressional Budget Office; staff of the Joint Committee on Taxation.

Notes: Figures for the nonelderly population include residents of the 50 states and the District of Columbia who are younger than 65.

　　　ACA = Affordable Care Act; CHIP = Children's Health Insurance Program; * = between -500,000 and zero; ** = between zero and 500,000.

a. Figures reflect average enrollment over the course of a year and include spouses and dependents covered under family policies; people reporting multiple sources of coverage are assigned a primary source.

b. "Other" includes Medicare; the changes under the ACA are almost entirely for nongroup coverage.

c. The uninsured population includes people who will be unauthorized immigrants and thus ineligible either for exchange subsidies or for most Medicaid benefits; people who will be ineligible for Medicaid because they live in a state that has chosen not to expand coverage; people who will be eligible for Medicaid but will choose not to enroll; and people who will not purchase insurance to which they have access through an employer, an exchange, or directly from an insurer.

d. The change in employment-based coverage is the net result of projected increases and decreases in offers of health insurance from employers and changes in enrollment by workers and their families.

e. Workers who would have to pay more than a specified share of their income (9.5 percent in 2014) for employment-based coverage could receive subsidies through an exchange.

f. Excludes coverage purchased directly from insurers outside of an exchange.

Figure 1.

Effects of the Affordable Care Act on Health Insurance Coverage, 2024

(Millions of nonelderly people)

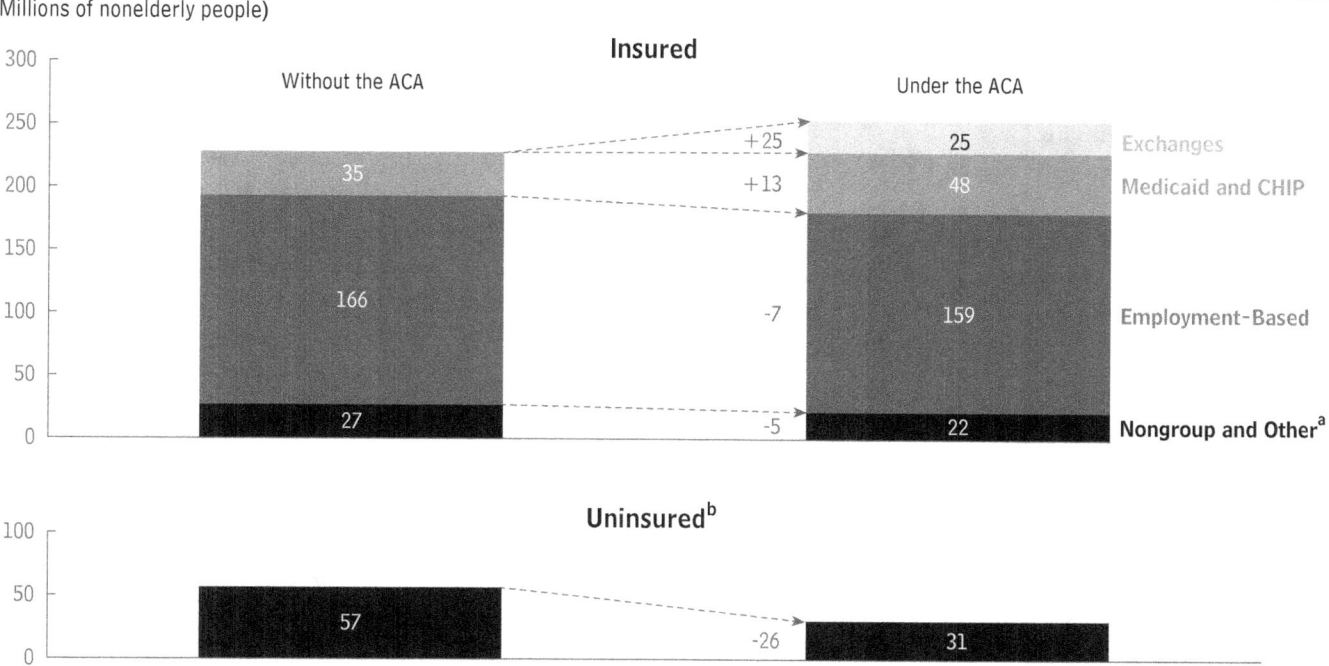

Sources: Congressional Budget Office; staff of the Joint Committee on Taxation.

Notes: The nonelderly population consists of residents of the 50 states and the District of Columbia who are younger than 65.

　　　ACA = Affordable Care Act; CHIP = Children's Health Insurance Program.

a.　"Other" includes Medicare; the changes under the ACA are almost entirely for nongroup coverage.

b.　The uninsured population includes people who will be unauthorized immigrants and thus ineligible either for exchange subsidies or for most Medicaid benefits; people who will be ineligible for Medicaid because they live in a state that has chosen not to expand coverage; people who will be eligible for Medicaid but will choose not to enroll; and people who will not purchase insurance to which they have access through an employer, an exchange, or directly from an insurer.

Despite the substantial projected increases in insurance coverage under the ACA, CBO and JCT estimate that in 2024, 31 million people, or roughly one in nine non-elderly U.S. residents, will be without health insurance (see Figure 1). In that year, about 30 percent of those uninsured people are expected to be unauthorized immigrants and thus ineligible either for exchange subsidies or for most Medicaid benefits; about 5 percent will be ineligible for Medicaid because they live in a state that has chosen not to expand coverage; about 20 percent will be eligible for Medicaid but will choose not to enroll; and the remaining 45 percent will not purchase insurance to which they have access through an employer, an exchange, or directly from an insurer.

Estimated Effects on Sources of Insurance Coverage and the Federal Budget

Most of the budgetary effects of the ACA's coverage provisions will stem from the subsidies for insurance purchased through the exchanges and from increased costs for Medicaid. That additional spending will be partially offset by penalty payments made by individuals and employers, by additional revenues resulting from the excise tax on high-premium insurance plans, and by the effects on income and payroll tax revenues and associated outlays stemming from a reduction in employment-based insurance coverage.

Coverage Through the Exchanges and Premiums and Subsidies for Such Coverage

Subsidies and related spending for insurance obtained through the exchanges constitute the largest share of the costs of the ACA's coverage provisions.

Coverage Through the Exchanges. CBO and JCT estimate that, over the course of calendar year 2014, an average of 6 million people will be covered by insurance obtained through the exchanges. The total number who will have such coverage at some points during the year is expected to be more than the average because some people will be covered for only part of the year.

Coverage through the exchanges will vary over the course of 2014 not only because of the increase during open enrollment in the first few months of the year but also because people who experience qualifying life events, such as the loss of employment-based insurance or the birth of a child, will be allowed to purchase coverage later in the year, and because some people will drop their exchange-based coverage as they become eligible for employment-based insurance. The estimate of 6 million people does not include people who enrolled through the exchanges but failed to pay their initial premiums, because they will not be covered; it also does not include people in any part of the year for which they lose coverage because of nonpayment of premiums.

Thus, CBO and JCT's estimate of 6 million people receiving such coverage in 2014 cannot be compared directly with the number of people who have enrolled through the exchanges as of any given date.[6] The number of people who will have coverage through the exchanges in 2014 will not be known precisely until after the year has ended.

CBO and JCT anticipate that coverage through the exchanges will increase substantially over time as more people respond to subsidies and to penalties for failure to obtain coverage. Coverage through the exchanges is projected to increase to an average of 13 million people in 2015, 24 million in 2016, and 25 million in each year between 2017 and 2024. Roughly three-quarters of those enrollees are expected to receive exchange subsidies.

Premiums for Exchange Coverage. CBO and JCT estimate that the average cost of individual policies for the second-lowest-cost "silver" plan in the exchanges—the benchmark for determining exchange subsidies—is about $3,800 in 2014.[7] That estimate represents a national average, and it reflects CBO and JCT's projections of the age, sex, health status, and geographic distribution of those who will obtain coverage through the exchanges in 2014. That benchmark premium is projected to rise slightly in 2015, to about $3,900, and then to rise more rapidly thereafter, reaching about $4,400 in 2016 and about $6,900 in 2024.[8] Thus, premiums are projected to increase by about 6 percent per year, on average, from 2016 to 2024. The current projection of the average premium for the benchmark silver plan in 2016 of about $4,400 is 15 percent below the comparable estimate of $5,200 published by CBO in November 2009.[9]

CBO and JCT anticipate that rising health care costs per person will continue to be the primary factor raising health insurance premiums over the next decade. Projecting the growth in health care spending per person always involves uncertainty, however, and it is particularly challenging in light of the recent slowdown in that growth that has been experienced by private insurers, as well as by the Medicare and Medicaid programs. Moreover,

---

6. See, for example, Department of Health and Human Services, Office of the Assistant Secretary for Planning and Evaluation, *Health Insurance Marketplace: March Enrollment Report for the Period: October 1, 2013–March 1, 2014*, ASPE Issue Brief (March 2014), http://go.usa.gov/Ksc4.

7. The size of the tax credit (or premium subsidy) that someone will receive will be based in part on the premium of the second-lowest-cost silver plan (which covers about 70 percent of the costs of covered benefits) offered through the exchange in which that person participates.

8. The average premium for all plans purchased through the exchanges will differ from the average for the benchmark plans because people can purchase plans with higher or lower actuarial value than the benchmark and with premiums that are more or less expensive than those for the second-lowest-cost silver plan.

9. See Congressional Budget Office, letter to the Honorable Evan Bayh providing an analysis of health insurance premiums under the Patient Protection and Affordable Care Act (November 30, 2009), www.cbo.gov/publication/41792. Similarly, the current projection of the average premium for a self-only policy in the employment-based market in 2016 of about $6,400 is 14 percent below the comparable estimate of $7,400 published by CBO in November 2009. See Congressional Budget Office, *Selected CBO Publications Related to Health Care Legislation, 2009–2010* (December 2010), p. 222, www.cbo.gov/publication/21993.

views differ on how much of the slowdown is attributable to the recession and its aftermath and how much to other factors. Exchange premiums will be affected not only by underlying growth in health care costs but also by changes in the average health status of enrollees, changes in federal programs that spread risk, and changes in plan characteristics. Those three factors are discussed in more detail below.

Effects of the Health Status of Exchange Enrollees. The premiums for policies sold in the exchanges will be influenced by the expected health status of enrollees in the exchanges, and CBO and JCT anticipate that exchange enrollees in the future will be healthier, on average, than the smaller number of people who are obtaining such coverage in 2014. Such an outcome would be expected if people who are less healthy are more eager to obtain insurance, and it would be consistent with enrollment and medical claims in Massachusetts after that state introduced subsidized exchanges in 2006.[10] That factor is expected to lower premiums in 2015 relative to those in 2014.

CBO and JCT do not expect any further significant shifts in the average health status of exchange enrollees after 2015 under current law. As a result, that factor is not expected to raise or lower premiums after 2015.

Actual exchange premiums for 2015 may differ from those CBO and JCT have projected because insurers could have different expectations of their costs for that year. For example, if enrollees in exchange plans in 2014 are significantly less healthy than insurers had expected, and their care therefore is significantly more costly, insurers could project notably higher costs in 2015 and charge correspondingly higher premiums in 2015 than in 2014. However, anecdotal reports to date have been mixed and provide no clear evidence that insurers have been substantially surprised by the health status of their enrollees. Moreover, CBO and JCT's projections are national averages, and premiums in some places in the country will probably be much higher or lower in 2015 than CBO and JCT have projected for the nation as a whole.

Effects of the Reinsurance Program. The premiums for policies sold in the exchanges also are affected by the reinsurance payments that the government will make to plans whose enrollees incur particularly high costs for medical care—that is, costs that are above a specified threshold and up to a certain maximum. The reinsurance program applies to all nongroup insurance that complies with the ACA's market and benefit standards and that is issued from 2014 through 2016, either within or outside of the exchanges. (For more information on the ACA's provisions governing the nongroup market, see Box 1.)

Under the reinsurance program, CBO and JCT project, the government will collect $10 billion in 2015, $6 billion in 2016, and $4 billion in 2017 (for insurance issued in 2014, 2015, and 2016) through a per-enrollee assessment on most private insurance plans, including self-insured plans and plans that are offered in the large-group market.[11] CBO and JCT expect that reinsurance payments scheduled for insurance provided in 2014 are large enough to have reduced exchange premiums this year by approximately 10 percent relative to what they would have been without the program. However, such payments will be significantly smaller for 2015 and 2016, and they will not occur for the years following. Therefore, that program is expected to have resulted in lower premiums in 2014, to reduce premiums by smaller amounts in 2015 and 2016 than in 2014, and to have no direct effect thereafter.

Effects of the Characteristics of Exchange Plans. The plans being offered through exchanges in 2014 appear to have, in general, lower payment rates for providers, narrower networks of providers, and tighter management of their subscribers' use of health care than employment-based plans do.[12] Those features allow insurers that offer plans through the exchanges to charge lower premiums (although they also make plans somewhat less attractive

---

10. See Amitabh Chandra, Jonathan Gruber, and Robin McKnight, "The Importance of the Individual Mandate—Evidence From Massachusetts," *New England Journal of Medicine* (January 2011), vol. 364, no. 4, pp. 293–295, http://tinyurl.com/496lfct. CBO analyzed unpublished data provided by the authors of that article.

11. Under reinsurance, an additional $5 billion will be collected from health insurance plans and deposited into the general fund of the U.S. Treasury. That amount is the same as the amount appropriated for the Early Retiree Reinsurance Program (which was in operation before 2014) and is not included here as part of the budgetary effects of the ACA's insurance coverage provisions.

12. See McKinsey & Company, *Exchanges Go Live: Early Trends in Exchange Dynamics* (October 2013), http://tinyurl.com/qd3kqfl, and *Emerging Exchange Dynamics: Temporary Turbulence or Sustainable Market Disruption?* (September 2013), http://tinyurl.com/og3tu9d.

Box 1.

Nongroup Health Plans Under the Affordable Care Act

Starting in 2014, companies that sell nongroup insurance plans, whether through the exchanges or not, must—in most cases—follow certain rules specified in the Affordable Care Act (ACA).[1] All new plans, for example, must cover a set of essential health benefits, and their premiums may not vary among enrollees on the basis of health. Insurers selling nongroup plans through the exchanges must offer at least one "silver" plan (with an actuarial value of 70 percent) and one "gold" plan (80 percent).[2] Insurers selling plans outside of the exchanges must follow the same system of "metal" tiers, ranging from 60 percent ("bronze") to 90 percent ("platinum"), but, unlike insurers in the exchanges, they are exempt from the requirement to offer at least one silver and one gold plan.[3] Plans must be available for anyone to purchase during specified annual open-enrollment periods and, outside of those periods, to anyone who experiences a qualifying life event, such as the birth of a child or a change in employment. States may impose additional requirements on insurers that offer nongroup coverage inside or outside of the exchanges.

Because of the uncertainty about average health care costs for people enrolling under the new rules governing the nongroup market, plans that comply with the ACA's rules are protected from some of the risk that they will attract enrollees whose health care costs will prove to be especially high.[4] The Congressional Budget Office (CBO) and the staff of the Joint Committee on Taxation (JCT) expect that people who purchase ACA-compliant plans outside of the exchanges would probably not have been eligible for subsidies had they obtained coverage through the exchanges and that many would have purchased coverage in the nongroup market in the absence of the ACA.

---

1. Nongroup plans are those sold to individuals and families rather than to employers or groups of people.

2. A plan's actuarial value is the share of costs for covered services that it would pay, on average, with a broadly representative group of people enrolled.

3. People under 30 years of age and those who qualify for certain exemptions from the individual mandate penalty also may purchase catastrophic coverage inside or outside of the exchanges. Such plans incorporate the ACA's set of essential health benefits, but they are not required to meet a minimum actuarial value of 60 percent. Catastrophic plans have a high deductible that is equal to the plan's out-of-pocket maximum and do not qualify for premium or cost-sharing subsidies, even when offered through the exchanges.

4. Among the federal safeguards that reduce the risk are the risk adjustment and reinsurance programs (which apply to all ACA-compliant nongroup plans), and risk corridors (which cover all exchange plans and also include certain plans offered outside the exchanges); for more discussion, see Congressional Budget Office, *The Budget and Economic Outlook: 2014 to 2024*, Appendix B (February 2014), www.cbo.gov/publication/45010.

Continued

---

to potential enrollees). As projected enrollment in exchange plans grows from an average of 6 million in 2014 to 24 million in 2016, CBO and JCT anticipate that many plans will not be able to sustain provider payment rates that are as low or networks that are as narrow as they appear to be in 2014. CBO and JCT expect that exchange plans will still have lower provider payment rates, more limited provider networks, and stricter management of care, on average, than employment-based plans but that the differences between employment-based plans and exchange plans will narrow as exchange enrollment increases. That pattern will put upward pressure on exchange premiums over the next couple of years, although CBO and JCT anticipate that the plans' characteristics will stabilize after 2016.

Subsidies for Exchange Coverage and Related Spending. Exchange subsidies depend both on benchmark premiums in the exchanges and on certain characteristics of enrollees, such as age, family size, geographic location, and income. CBO and JCT project that the average subsidy will be $4,410 in 2014, that it will decline to $4,250 in 2015, and that it will then rise each year to reach $7,170 in 2024 (see Table 2 on page 4).[13] The projected decrease from 2014 to 2015 stems from the small projected increase in premiums in 2015 and a shift in the income of people who are projected to enroll in the

---

13. The average exchange subsidy per subsidized enrollee includes premium subsidies and cost-sharing subsidies and thus may exceed the average benchmark premium in the exchanges.

Under certain limited circumstances, insurers are allowed to continue to sell policies that do not comply with the ACA's rules. Such noncompliant policies, for example, might not cover all of the essential benefits specified in the ACA, might have an actuarial value of less than 60 percent, or might charge lower premiums for people in better health.[5] Those limited circumstances include the following:

■ Some policies can be "grandfathered" in. Policies that were in effect in March 2010 and that have been maintained continuously without substantial changes in benefits or in costs to enrollees are exempt from most of the ACA's rules.

■ Some states permitted insurers to allow enrollees to renew policies that did not comply with certain market and benefit rules for 2014 so long as the policy year began before January 1, 2014.

■ Some policies can qualify under what is known as transitional relief. In November 2013, the Administration announced that states could accept renewals of noncompliant policies for a policy year starting between January 1, 2014, and October 1, 2014. In March 2014, that transitional

---

5. Insurers may also sell other policies that are service specific (including dental and vision), that cover accidental injury or specific diseases, or that are in effect for only a short time; such plans do not, on their own, count as providing minimum essential coverage under the ACA. Such plans are not included in CBO and JCT's estimates of coverage under the ACA.

relief was extended for two more years. (More detail on recent administrative actions that affect noncompliant plans is provided in "Availability of Noncompliant Plans" in the main text.)

CBO and JCT estimate that relatively few people will be enrolled in noncompliant nongroup plans. The agencies project that, under the ACA, in 2014 about 2 million people will purchase noncompliant plans; they anticipate that enrollment in such plans will decline to negligible numbers by 2016. They also project that enrollment in nongroup plans *through the exchanges* will average 6 million people in 2014, 13 million in 2015, and 24 million or 25 million each year thereafter, and that roughly 5 million people will enroll in ACA-compliant plans *outside of the exchanges* each year from 2014 through 2024. That last estimate is especially uncertain because information on the number of people who have purchased coverage in the nongroup market in past years is incomplete and varies widely by data source.

In the absence of the ACA, 9 million to 10 million people would have enrolled in nongroup coverage each year from 2014 through 2024, CBO and JCT estimate. With roughly 5 million people expected to enroll in nongroup plans in years after 2015 under the ACA (excluding those people who purchase policies through the exchanges), that number will be 4 million to 5 million lower under the ACA than the number projected in the absence of the law (see the change in coverage labeled "Nongroup and other coverage" in Table 2 of the main text).

---

exchanges in 2015 compared with those enrolling in 2014. The increases after 2015 stem largely from the projected increase in premiums.

CBO and JCT estimate that subsidies provided through the exchanges and related spending will total $17 billion in 2014. That estimate is uncertain in part because the number of people who will have such coverage is not yet known and in part because detailed information on the demographics and family income of the people who have such coverage—and on the subsidies they will receive—is not yet available. Over the 10 years from 2015 to 2024, exchange subsidies and related spending are projected to total $1,032 billion, distributed as follows:

■ Outlays of $726 billion and a reduction in revenues of $129 billion for premium assistance tax credits (to cover a portion of eligible individuals' and families' health insurance premiums), which sum to $855 billion (see Table 3);[14]

---

14. The subsidies for health insurance premiums are structured as refundable tax credits; following the usual procedures for such credits, the portions that exceed taxpayers' income tax liabilities are classified as outlays in CBO's baseline projections, and the portions that reduce tax payments are classified as reductions in revenues.

Table 3.

Enrollment in, and Budgetary Effects of, Health Insurance Exchanges

	2014	2015	2016	2017	2018	2019	2020	2021	2022	2023	2024	Total, 2015– 2024
	Exchange Enrollment (Millions of nonelderly people, by calendar year)[a]											
Individually Purchased Coverage												
Subsidized	5	10	19	19	20	19	19	19	19	19	19	n.a.
Unsubsidized[b]	1	3	5	6	6	6	6	6	6	6	6	n.a.
Total	6	13	24	25	25	25	25	25	25	25	25	n.a.
Employment-Based Coverage Purchased Through Exchanges[b]	2	3	3	4	4	4	4	4	4	4	4	n.a.
	Budgetary Effects (Billions of dollars, by fiscal year)											
Changes in Mandatory Spending												
Outlays for premium credits	10	23	51	65	71	75	79	84	89	93	95	726
Cost-sharing subsidies	3	7	13	16	17	18	19	20	21	22	22	175
Exchange grants to states	2	2	1	*	*	0	0	0	0	0	0	2
Payments for risk adjustment, reinsurance, and risk corridors	0	18	19	22	15	17	18	19	19	20	19	186
Total	15	50	84	104	103	109	116	123	129	134	137	1,089
Changes in Revenues												
Reductions in revenues from premium credits	-2	-5	-10	-12	-13	-14	-14	-15	-15	-15	-15	-129
Collections for risk adjustment, reinsurance, and risk corridors	0	19	18	22	15	17	18	19	19	20	19	186
Total	-2	14	7	10	2	3	4	4	4	5	5	56
Net Increase in the Deficit From Exchange Subsidies and Related Spending	17	36	77	94	101	107	112	119	125	129	132	1,032
Memorandum:												
Total Subsidies Through Premium Credits (Billions of dollars, by fiscal year)	12	29	62	78	84	89	93	99	104	108	110	855
Total Exchange Subsidies (Billions of dollars, by calendar year)	21	42	89	95	104	108	114	121	127	130	133	1,064
Average Exchange Subsidy per Subsidized Enrollee (Dollars, by calendar year)	4,410	4,250	4,830	4,930	5,300	5,570	5,880	6,220	6,580	6,890	7,170	n.a.

Sources: Congressional Budget Office; staff of the Joint Committee on Taxation.

Note: n.a. = not applicable; * = between zero and $500 million.

a. Figures reflect average enrollment over the course of a year and include spouses and dependents covered under family policies. Figures for the nonelderly population include residents of the 50 states and the District of Columbia who are younger than 65.

b. Excludes coverage purchased directly from insurers outside of an exchange.

- Outlays of $175 billion for cost-sharing subsidies (to reduce out-of-pocket payments for low-income enrollees);

- Outlays of $2 billion for grants to states for operating exchanges; and

- Outlays and revenues each totaling $186 billion related to payments and collections for risk adjustment, reinsurance, and risk corridors (having no net budgetary effect).

The ACA's provisions for risk adjustment, reinsurance, and risk corridors generate payments by the federal government to insurers and collections by the federal government from insurers that reflect differences in health status and costs among insurers' enrollees.[15] CBO treats the payments as outlays and the collections as revenues and projects that, over the 2015–2024 period, risk adjustment payments and collections will total $156 billion each and reinsurance payments and collections will total $20 billion each. Over that same period, CBO estimates, risk corridor payments from the federal government to health insurers will total $9 billion and the corresponding collections from insurers will amount to $9 billion, thus having no net budgetary effect. (The section below, "Changes From Previous Estimates," discusses the changes in those figures from the previous projection and the reasons for the changes.)

Enrollment in Medicaid and CHIP and the Federal Cost of Such Coverage

CBO and JCT project that substantially more people will be enrolled in Medicaid and CHIP than would have been the case in the absence of the ACA—7 million more in calendar year 2014, 11 million more in 2015, and 12 million to 13 million more people in each year between 2016 and 2024 (see Table 2 on page 4).[16] Some of those additional enrollees will be people who become eligible for Medicaid because of the ACA's coverage expansion; others will be people who would have been eligible for Medicaid or CHIP in the absence of the ACA but would not have enrolled. CBO expects that the ACA's individual mandate, increased outreach, and new

opportunities to enroll in those programs through exchanges will increase enrollment among people who were previously eligible.

The anticipated increase in Medicaid enrollment after 2014 reflects the expectation that more people in states that have already expanded Medicaid eligibility will enroll in the program and that more states will expand Medicaid eligibility. Those increases will be partially offset by lower enrollment in CHIP, starting in 2016; in CBO's baseline, funding projected for that program is lower in 2016 and following years than is anticipated for the next two years.[17]

As with exchange enrollment, the projected figures represent averages over the course of those years and differ from estimates of enrollment at any particular point during a year. CBO and JCT expect that, once the ACA is fully phased in, enrollment in Medicaid and CHIP will vary over the course of each year. Unlike exchange plans, which offer limited annual open-enrollment periods, Medicaid and CHIP are open to eligible people at any time. As a result, people move in and out of coverage for many reasons, including a change in their need for health care; a change in their awareness of the availability of coverage; or a change in circumstances that affects program eligibility, such as a change in income or the birth of a

---

15. For more details, see Congressional Budget Office, *The Budget and Economic Outlook: 2014 to 2024*, Appendix B (February 2014), www.cbo.gov/publication/45010.

16. Early in April 2014, the Department of Health and Human Services issued the fifth in a series of monthly reports on state Medicaid and CHIP enrollment, providing a preliminary estimate of 3 million additional Medicaid and CHIP enrollees at the end of February in 46 states (compared with enrollment in the months before the ACA's coverage expansions began). That number is noted to include people who were newly eligible for Medicaid because of the ACA's coverage expansion as well as those who were eligible for Medicaid and CHIP in the absence of the ACA but would not have signed up, and those who were re-enrolling. It does not, however, include new enrollees who applied for Medicaid through federally facilitated marketplaces. See Centers for Medicare & Medicaid Services, *Medicaid & CHIP: February 2014 Monthly Applications, Eligibility Determinations, and Enrollment Report* (April 4, 2014), http://go.usa.gov/k2az (PDF, 688 KB).

17. Annual spending for CHIP is projected to reach $12.5 billion in 2015—the final year in which the program is fully funded under current law. Under the rules governing baseline projections for expiring programs, CBO projects funding for CHIP after 2015 at an annualized amount of about $6 billion. For more details about the CHIP baseline, see Congressional Budget Office, "Children's Health Insurance Program Spending and Enrollment Detail for CBO's April 2014 Baseline," www.cbo.gov/publication/45229.

child. Therefore, the number of people who receive coverage through Medicaid and CHIP in any year will not generally be known precisely until well after the year has ended and state enrollment data have become available.

Furthermore, it will never be possible to determine how many people who sign up for Medicaid would have been eligible but not enrolled in the absence of the ACA. The number of people who sign up who are newly eligible *can* be determined because states that expand coverage under the act will report the number of enrollees who became eligible as a result of that expansion in order to receive the additional federal funding that will be provided for such enrollees. But there will be no way to tell whether people who sign up who would have been eligible without the ACA would, or would not, have enrolled anyway.

CBO and JCT estimate that the added costs to the federal government for Medicaid and CHIP attributable to the ACA will be $20 billion in 2014 and will total $792 billion for the 2015–2024 period (see Table 1 on page 2).

The extent of the expansion of insurance coverage through all sources in 2014 as a result of the ACA will not be clear until more time has elapsed and more data are available. The government is collecting data on the number of people who sign up for coverage in the exchanges, Medicaid, and CHIP; moreover, the ACA requires additional information on coverage to be reported by employers and health insurance providers. In addition, CBO and JCT monitor various sources of survey data—including large, federally sponsored surveys of households and employers as well as smaller, privately funded surveys that use telephone and online questionnaires.[18] However, some data will be available only after a delay—anywhere from a few months to a few years. Moreover, differences must be reconciled within and among data sets to arrive at a clear picture of changes in overall insurance coverage and the sources of such coverage.

---

18. Among the sources that CBO and JCT will consult in their analyses of the ACA's effects are the Department of Health and Human Services' National Health Interview Survey, results from Gallup polls, the Urban Institute's Health Reform Monitoring Survey, and RAND's American Life Panel Survey. Also, more detailed information on changes in coverage by family income will come later from the Census Bureau's Current Population Survey and the Department of Health and Human Services' Medical Expenditure Panel Survey.

Tax Credits for Small Employers

Under the ACA, certain small employers are eligible to receive tax credits to defray the cost of providing health insurance to their employees. CBO and JCT project that those tax credits will total $1 billion in 2014 and $15 billion over the 2015–2024 period.

Penalty Payments by Uninsured People

Beginning in 2014, the ACA requires most legal residents of the United States to obtain health insurance or pay a penalty. People who do not obtain coverage will pay the greater of two amounts: either a flat dollar penalty per adult in a family, rising from $95 in 2014 to $695 in 2016 and indexed to inflation thereafter (the penalty for a child is half the amount, and an overall cap will apply to family payments); or a percentage of a household's adjusted gross income in excess of the income threshold for mandatory tax-filing—a share that will rise from 1.0 percent in 2014 to 2.5 percent in 2016 and subsequent years (also subject to a cap). CBO and JCT estimate that such payments from individuals will total $46 billion over the 2015–2024 period.

Some people, such as unauthorized immigrants, are not subject to the requirement to obtain health insurance. Other people face the requirement but are exempt from the penalty, for example, because their income is low enough that they do not file income tax returns, their income is below 138 percent of federal poverty guidelines and they are ineligible for Medicaid because their state did not expand the program, they are members of an Indian tribe, or their premiums would exceed a specified share of their income (8 percent in 2014 and indexed for inflation over time). Certain other exemptions are described below in the section "Regulations and Other Administrative Actions."

Penalty Payments by Employers

Beginning in 2015, certain large employers who do not offer health insurance that meets specified standards will pay a penalty if they have full-time employees who receive a subsidy through an exchange. The specified standards involve affordability and the share of the cost of covered benefits paid by the insurance plan.[19] Employers with at least 50 full-time-equivalent (FTE) employees will generally be subject to that requirement. In 2015

---

19. To meet the standards, the cost to the employee for self-only coverage must not exceed a specified share of income (9.5 percent in 2014 and indexed over time), and the plan must pay at least 60 percent of the cost of covered benefits.

only, however, employers with at least 50 but fewer than 100 FTE employees will be exempt from the requirement if they certify that they have not made certain reductions to health insurance coverage or reduced their number of FTE employees to avoid the penalties. (Recent changes to this aspect of the ACA are discussed below in "Employers' Responsibilities in 2015.") CBO and JCT estimate that penalty payments by employers will total $139 billion over the 2015–2024 period.

Excise Tax on High-Premium Insurance Plans

According to CBO and JCT's estimates, federal revenues will increase by $120 billion over the 2015–2024 period because of the excise tax on high-premium insurance plans. Roughly one-quarter of that increase stems from excise tax receipts, and roughly three-quarters is from the effects on revenues of changes in employees' taxable compensation and, to a lesser extent, in employers' deductible expenses. In particular, CBO and JCT anticipate that many employers and workers will shift to health plans with premiums that are below the specified thresholds to avoid paying the tax, resulting generally in higher taxable wages for affected workers.

Other Effects on Revenues and Outlays

The ACA also will affect federal tax revenues because fewer people will have employment-based health insurance and thus more of their income will take the form of taxable wages. CBO and JCT project that, as a result of the ACA, between 7 million and 8 million fewer people will have employment-based insurance each year from 2016 through 2024 than would have been the case in the absence of the ACA. That difference is the net result of projected increases and decreases in offers of health insurance from employers and of choices about enrollment by active workers, early retirees (people under the age of 65 at retirement), and their families.

In 2019, for example, an estimated 13 million people who would have enrolled in employment-based coverage in the absence of the ACA will not have an offer of such coverage under the ACA; an estimated 3 million people who would have enrolled in employment-based coverage will have such an offer but will choose not to enroll. Some of those 16 million people are expected to gain coverage through some other source; others will forgo health insurance. Those decreases in employment-based coverage will be partially offset, however. About 8 million people who would not have had employment-based coverage in the absence of the ACA are expected to receive

such coverage under the ACA; they will either take up an offer of coverage they would have received anyway or take up a new offer. Some of those enrollees would have been uninsured in the absence of the ACA.

Because of the net reduction in employment-based coverage, the share of workers' pay that takes the form of nontaxable benefits (such as health insurance premiums) will be smaller—and the share that takes the form of taxable wages will be larger—than would otherwise have been the case. That shift in compensation will boost federal tax receipts. Partially offsetting those added receipts will be an estimated $7 billion increase in Social Security benefits that will arise from the higher wages paid to workers. All told, CBO and JCT project, those effects will reduce federal budget deficits by $152 billion over the 2015–2024 period.

Changes From Previous Estimates

CBO and JCT currently estimate that the insurance coverage provisions of the ACA will have a smaller budgetary cost than those agencies estimated in February 2014.[20] CBO and JCT now estimate that the net cost to the federal government of those provisions for fiscal year 2014 will be $36 billion, $5 billion less than the previous estimate of $41 billion, and that the net cost for the 2015–2024 period will be $1,383 billion, $104 billion (or 7 percent) below the previous estimate of $1,487 billion (see Table 4).

CBO and JCT have updated their baseline estimates of the budgetary effects of the ACA's insurance coverage provisions many times since that legislation was enacted in March 2010. As time has passed, the period spanned by the estimates has changed, but a year-by-year comparison shows that CBO and JCT's estimates of the net budgetary impact of the ACA's insurance coverage provisions have decreased, on balance, over the past four years.

The first part of this section describes the factors that led to changes in CBO and JCT's estimates since February 2014, the second part summarizes the changes themselves, and the third part discusses changes in projected budgetary effects since the legislation was enacted in March 2010.

---

20. See Congressional Budget Office, *The Budget and Economic Outlook: 2014 to 2024*, Appendix B (February 2014), www.cbo.gov/publication/45010.

Table 4.

Comparison of CBO and JCT's Current and Previous Estimates of the Effects of the Insurance Coverage Provisions of the Affordable Care Act

	February 2014 Baseline	April 2014 Baseline	Difference
	Change in Insurance Coverage Under the ACA in 2024 (Millions of nonelderly people, by calendar year)[a]		
Insurance Exchanges	24	25	*
Medicaid and CHIP	13	13	1
Employment-Based Coverage[b]	-7	-7	-1
Nongroup and Other Coverage[c]	-5	-5	*
Uninsured[d]	-25	-26	-1
	Effects on the Cumulative Federal Deficit, 2015 to 2024[e] (Billions of dollars)		
Exchange Subsidies and Related Spending[f]	1,197	1,032	-164
Medicaid and CHIP Outlays	792	792	**
Small-Employer Tax Credits[g]	15	15	**
Gross Cost of Coverage Provisions	2,004	1,839	-165
Penalty Payments by Uninsured People	-52	-46	6
Penalty Payments by Employers[g]	-151	-139	12
Excise Tax on High-Premium Insurance Plans[g]	-108	-120	-12
Other Effects on Revenues and Outlays[h]	-206	-152	54
Net Cost of Coverage Provisions	**1,487**	**1,383**	**-104**
Memorandum:			
Net Collections and Payments for Risk Adjustment, Reinsurance, and Risk Corridors[i]	-8	0	8

Sources: Congressional Budget Office; staff of the Joint Committee on Taxation.

Note: ACA = Affordable Care Act; CHIP = Children's Health Insurance Program; * = between zero and 500,000;
** = between -$500 million and $500 million.

a. Figures for the nonelderly population include residents of the 50 states and the District of Columbia who are younger than 65.

b. The change in employment-based coverage is the net result of projected increases and decreases in offers of health insurance from employers and changes in enrollment by workers and their families.

c. "Other" includes Medicare; the changes under the ACA are almost entirely for nongroup coverage.

d. The uninsured population includes people who will be unauthorized immigrants and thus ineligible either for exchange subsidies or for most Medicaid benefits; people who will be ineligible for Medicaid because they live in a state that has chosen not to expand coverage; people who will be eligible for Medicaid but will choose not to enroll; and people who will not purchase insurance to which they have access through an employer, an exchange, or directly from an insurer.

e. Positive numbers indicate an increase in the deficit; negative numbers indicate a decrease in the deficit. They also exclude effects on the deficit of other provisions of the ACA that are not related to insurance coverage, and they exclude federal administrative costs subject to appropriation.

f. Includes spending for exchange grants to states and net collections and payments for risk adjustment, reinsurance, and risk corridors (see "Memorandum").

g. These effects on the deficit include the associated effects of changes in taxable compensation on revenues.

h. Consists mainly of the effects of changes in taxable compensation on revenues.

i. These effects are included in "Exchange Subsidies and Related Spending."

Factors That Led to Changes in the Estimates Since February 2014

The reductions in estimated federal costs are the net result of a combination of factors. The current projections:

- Incorporate the economic forecast that CBO published in February 2014; because the projections of the effects of the ACA's coverage provisions published in February were partial and preliminary, they did not incorporate the economic forecast published by CBO at that time.

- Incorporate further analyses by CBO and JCT of exchange premiums and the characteristics of exchange plans.

- Include revisions to estimates of the number of early retirees with employment-based coverage under the ACA.

- Account for regulations and other administrative actions that were put in place between early December 2013 and the end of March 2014.

Because of the way that various factors interact, it is not possible to isolate the effects of changes in individual factors on specific components of the budgetary effects.

Changes From Incorporating the February 2014 Economic Forecast.

In CBO's most recent economic forecast, published in February 2014, the agency revised its projections of various economic factors that will affect the number of people who will be eligible for subsidized insurance coverage under the ACA.[21] Changes in estimates of labor force participation, wages and salaries, and population had the largest effects on projections of eligibility for subsidized coverage.

The projected labor force participation rate among people younger than age 65 is lower throughout the next decade than it was in the forecast CBO published in 2013. In 2020, for example, CBO now anticipates that this participation rate will be 75.9 percent, compared with the 76.5 percent it projected previously.[22] The

downward revision stems from a variety of factors, and it results in a slightly larger projection of the number of people who will be eligible for Medicaid, CHIP, and subsidies in the exchanges.

Wages and salaries also are projected to be lower through most of the next decade than they were in CBO's previous forecast—by between 4 percent and 5 percent, for example, from 2018 through 2023. The result of that and other changes to the income projections, including changes to the projected distribution of income, is a slight increase in Medicaid eligibility and a slight decrease in eligibility for premium subsidies.

CBO revised its projection of the total population under the age of 65 as a result of incorporating recently available information from the 2010 decennial census. Under the revised projection, the nonelderly population during the years from 2014 to 2024 is 2 million to 4 million people smaller than it was in the previous projection. Taken together with information on the employment-based health insurance market, that change resulted most notably in a downward revision of CBO and JCT's projection of the number of people without insurance in the absence of the ACA during the early years of the coming decade.

In addition, CBO and JCT made a related technical adjustment on the basis of a more detailed analysis of survey data. The agencies altered their projections of the age mix of people who would have been without insurance in the absence of the ACA, reducing the projected share of children in that group. As discussed later, that change affects CBO and JCT's projection of the number of people who will enroll in Medicaid and CHIP under the ACA.

Changes in Estimated Exchange Premiums.

In the February 2014 projections, CBO and JCT reduced their estimate of exchange premiums for 2014. However, no changes were made to premium projections for later years because the February update was partial and preliminary. The current update of the baseline incorporates the results of additional analyses of the premiums charged for

---

21. See Congressional Budget Office, *The Budget and Economic Outlook: 2014 to 2024*, Chapter 2 (February 2014), www.cbo.gov/publication/45010.

22. CBO regularly publishes forecasts of labor force participation for people of all ages, but not for people under age 65. Those published rates show a similar revision.

2014, resulting in changes to the estimates for 2014 and for later years.

A crucial factor in the current revision was an analysis of the characteristics of plans offered through the exchanges in 2014. Previously, CBO and JCT had expected that those plans' characteristics would closely resemble the characteristics of employment-based plans throughout the projection period. However, the plans being offered through the exchanges this year appear to have, in general, lower payment rates for providers, narrower networks of providers, and tighter management of their subscribers' use of health care than employment-based plans do.

CBO and JCT anticipate that, as enrollment in the exchanges rises, the differences between employment-based plans and exchange plans will narrow. Therefore, projected premiums during the next few years were revised downward more than were premiums for the later years of the coming decade.

The lower exchange premiums and revisions to the other characteristics of insurance plans that are incorporated into CBO and JCT's current estimates have small effects on the agencies' projections of exchange enrollment. Although lower premiums will tend to increase enrollment, narrower networks and more tightly managed benefits will tend to reduce the attractiveness of plans and thereby decrease enrollment. The net effect on projected enrollment in the exchanges is small.

Lower premiums also have the effect of reducing the federal cost of exchange subsidies. The current estimate of the average subsidy for 2014 is about $300 (or 6 percent) less than the estimate in the February 2014 baseline, and the estimate for 2024 is about $1,200 (or 14 percent) below the earlier projection. The reductions in subsidies relative to the previous baseline are smaller for 2014 than for later years because, in February, CBO and JCT updated their estimates of exchange premiums and subsidies for 2014 but did not make changes to those estimates for 2015 or later years.

Changes in the Estimates of the Number of People With Employment-Based Coverage. CBO and JCT have revised their projections both of the number of people and of the groups of people who will obtain coverage from current or former employers. As a result of several technical modeling adjustments, the agencies' estimates

of active workers and their dependents with such coverage have been revised upward by about 1 million people in most years. At the same time, CBO and JCT have revised downward their estimates of the number of non-elderly retirees with health insurance from a previous employer. Part of that revision stems from a reevaluation of the decline in retiree coverage over the past decade in the absence of the ACA. Another part is attributable to an assessment that more employers than previously thought will decide not to offer retiree coverage under the ACA—both because of the availability of the exchanges and other new sources of coverage and because they face no penalty for declining to offer coverage to retirees. Those considerations led CBO and JCT to reduce their projections—by about 2 million people in most years—of the number of early retirees and their dependents who will be covered by employment-based health insurance under the ACA and to increase their projections of the number who will enroll in the exchanges.

The net effect of the upward revision in coverage of active workers and the downward revision in coverage of retired workers is a downward revision—by about 1 million people for most years—in the projection of the number of people with employment-based coverage under the ACA.

CBO and JCT anticipate that the effect on tax revenues from employers' declining to offer coverage to retirees will be significantly smaller than the effect of such a decision regarding active employees. The decision of employers not to offer health insurance to active employees generally boosts federal revenues in two ways—by raising employees' taxable compensation and by raising penalties paid by employers who are subject to the ACA's requirements concerning employment-based coverage. For retirees' coverage, however, a smaller portion of premium costs tends to be excluded from taxable income, so replacing retirees' coverage with an increase in other forms of employee compensation generates less additional tax revenue than would a similar change involving active employees. Also, as noted, employers face no penalty for not offering coverage to retirees.

Regulations and Other Administrative Actions. The Administration has released several proposed and final regulations and announced other actions regarding implementation of the ACA since early December 2013, when CBO's February 2014 baseline projections were completed. The implications for CBO and JCT's projections of four significant actions are described here.

Employers' Responsibilities in 2015. Under the ACA, certain employers with 50 or more FTE employees that do not offer health insurance coverage that meets the standards specified in law will be subject to penalties. That requirement initially was to take effect in January 2014, but in July 2013 the Administration delayed the requirement by one year and set it to take effect in January 2015.[23] That delay was incorporated into CBO and JCT's February 2014 projections.

In February 2014, the Department of the Treasury issued a final regulation providing additional transitional relief to employers. Employers with at least 50 but fewer than 100 FTE employees will be exempt from the employer requirement in 2015 if they certify that they have not made certain reductions to health insurance coverage or reduced their number of FTE employees to avoid the penalties. That final regulation also provided for a one-year relaxation of a related coverage requirement for employers subject to the requirement. That change took two forms. First, in 2015, those employers must offer coverage to at least 70 percent of their full-time employees—rather than the 95 percent specified in the proposed regulation. Second, in 2015, employers with at least 100 FTE employees are permitted to exclude the first 80 full-time employees from the penalty calculation (rather than the first 30 full-time employees, as will be the case in subsequent years).

That additional transitional relief was not included in the February 2014 projections. Incorporating the effects of that regulation led CBO and JCT to estimate slightly lower enrollment in employment-based coverage in 2015 and to estimate slightly less in revenues from penalties paid by employers in 2016. (Because penalties are collected the year after they are assessed, the 2015 delay will reduce collections in 2016.)

Availability of Noncompliant Plans. Under the ACA, health insurance policies sold by insurers must—in most cases—comply with certain rules, among them a prohibition on adjusting premiums on the basis of an applicant's health status and a requirement that insurers in the nongroup and small-group markets offer plans to all

applicants that cover certain essential health benefits and that pay a specified minimum share of the cost of covered benefits. Those requirements apply to plans sold both within and outside of the exchanges. (For more information on the nongroup market under the ACA, see Box 1 on page 8.) However, in March 2014, the Department of Health and Human Services announced that, through October 1, 2016, state insurance commissioners could permit health insurers to re-enroll individuals and small businesses in existing plans that do not comply with certain market and benefit rules that took effect in 2014, allowing such coverage to continue through September 2017. That announcement extended an action announced in November 2013 that permitted the renewal of noncompliant policies through October 1, 2014 (extending that coverage through September 2015).

CBO and JCT estimate that the March 2014 announcement will slightly reduce enrollment in ACA-compliant plans because some people will take advantage of this option by renewing their coverage in noncompliant plans. CBO and JCT also estimate that the March announcement will slightly reduce spending for exchange subsidies because some people who would have enrolled in a subsidized plan through the exchanges will instead renew coverage in noncompliant plans (which cannot be sold through the exchanges and are not subsidized). In addition, the lower premiums that small employers and self-employed people are likely to pay for noncompliant plans will generate a small amount of additional tax revenues because of those enrollees' resulting increased taxable income.

CBO and JCT expect that people who renew noncompliant plans will be healthier, on average, than people who enroll in ACA-compliant plans, leading to slightly higher medical claims per enrollee among ACA-compliant plans. However, CBO and JCT expect that such adjustments will have a negligible effect on average premiums in exchange plans because the number of people who re-enroll in noncompliant plans will probably be small relative to total enrollment in exchange plans.

Risk Corridors. The ACA established several programs to reduce the risk of financial losses faced by insurers. Under the temporary risk corridor program, the government will make payments during the next few years to companies that offer individual and small-group plans sold on the exchanges (and will make payments for certain plans sold outside of the exchanges if the plans are substantially the

---

23. For an estimate of the budgetary effects of that delay, see Congressional Budget Office, letter to the Honorable Paul Ryan providing an analysis of the Administration's announced delay of certain requirements under the Affordable Care Act (July 30, 2013), www.cbo.gov/publication/44465.

same as plans sold by the same carriers within the exchanges) when actual costs for medical claims exceed expected costs by certain percentages. At the same time, the government will receive payments from those plans whose actual costs for medical claims fall short of their expected costs by certain percentages.[24]

In March 2014, the Department of Health and Human Services issued a final regulation stating that its implementation of the risk corridor program will result in equal payments to and from the government, and thus will have no net budgetary effect. CBO believes that the Administration has sufficient flexibility to ensure that payments to insurers will approximately equal payments from insurers to the federal government, and thus that the program will have no net budgetary effect over the three years of its operation. (Previously, CBO had estimated that the risk corridor program would yield net budgetary savings of $8 billion.)

Hardship Exemption. In December 2013, the Department of Health and Human Services announced that it was allowing people whose nongroup plans were canceled by their insurers for 2014 to apply for a hardship waiver that would allow them either to remain uninsured without paying a penalty or to purchase lower-cost catastrophic coverage (plans with particularly high out-of-pocket costs for which most people would not ordinarily be eligible under the ACA).[25] In March 2014, the Department of Health and Human Services announced that this hardship waiver would be extended until October 1, 2016.[26]

People who apply for this hardship waiver will need to verify that they had been covered by a health insurance plan that was canceled. Because CBO and JCT expect that most of the people whose plans have been canceled will seek alternative sources of coverage rather than become uninsured, the agencies expect that this additional hardship exemption will have a negligible

effect on the amount of penalties collected from uninsured people. In addition, CBO and JCT expect that, for three reasons, a very small number of people who are permitted to enroll in a catastrophic plan will actually do so: Catastrophic plans have lower actuarial value than other types of coverage, people who enroll in catastrophic plans are ineligible for exchange subsidies, and CBO and JCT expect that many people either obtained coverage from another source for 2014 before the announcement or were unaware of that option at the time they sought coverage.

Changes in the Estimates Since February 2014

CBO and JCT currently estimate that the insurance coverage provisions of the ACA will have a net cost over the 2015–2024 period that is $104 billion less than the agencies estimated in February 2014. The difference stems from the following changes in estimates of the government's spending and collections (see Figure 2 on page 19 and Table 4 on page 14):

■ A reduction of $165 billion (or 8 percent) in the gross cost of the coverage provisions, almost entirely because exchange subsidies and related spending are now projected to cost $1,032 billion, compared with the previous estimate of $1,197 billion; and

■ A partially offsetting net reduction of $61 billion in savings as a result of lower expected penalty payments from uninsured people and employers, higher expected revenue resulting from the excise tax on certain high-premium employment-based insurance plans, and lower savings from other budgetary effects (mostly decreases in tax revenues).

Exchange Subsidies and Related Spending. CBO and JCT have not changed their previous estimate of the number of people who will purchase coverage through the exchanges in 2014. After 2014, however, CBO and JCT's estimates of enrollment are slightly higher than those in the previous projection—by less than 1 million people annually for most years. That increase has various origins, as discussed above, including lower expected premiums in the exchanges and less expected employment-based coverage for early retirees, both of which would increase the number of people purchasing insurance through the exchanges. Partially offsetting those factors are a slight downward shift in the expected income distribution (which reduces the number of people anticipated to be eligible for exchange subsidies) and

24. For more information, see Congressional Budget Office, *The Budget and Economic Outlook: 2014 to 2024*, Appendix B (February 2014), www.cbo.gov/publication/45010.

25. See Centers for Medicare & Medicaid Services, "Options Available for Consumers With Cancelled Policies" (December 19, 2013), http://go.usa.gov/KHTw (PDF, 110 KB).

26. See Centers for Medicare & Medicaid Services, "Insurance Standards Bulletin Series—Extension of Transitional Policy Through October 1, 2016" (March 5, 2014), http://go.usa.gov/KHbh (PDF, 148 KB).

Figure 2.

Budgetary Effects of the Insurance Coverage Provisions of the Affordable Care Act, 2015 to 2024

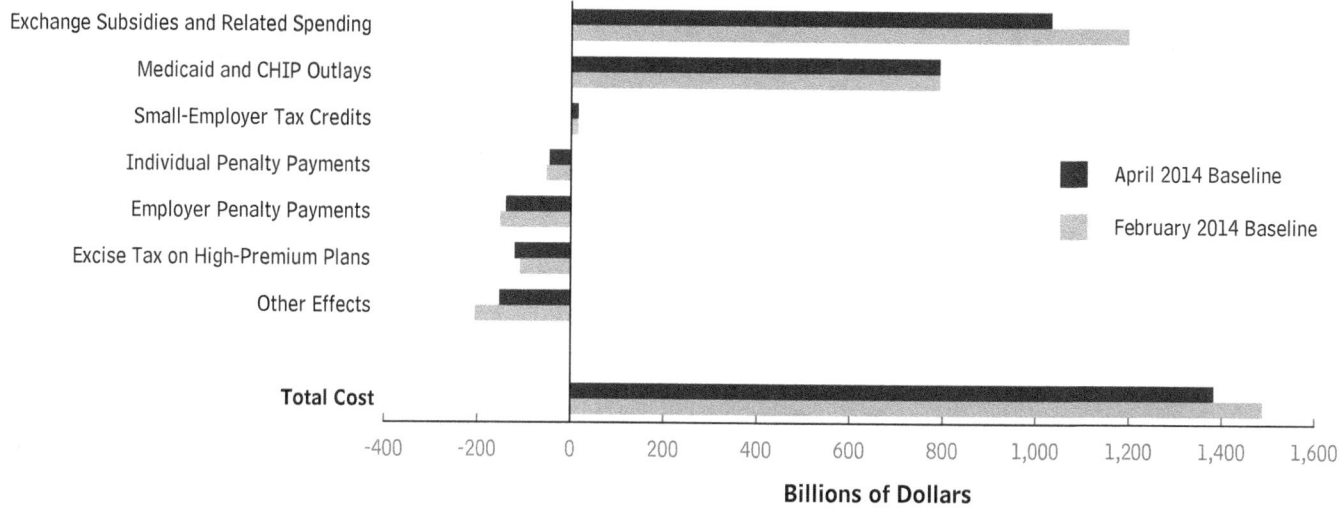

Sources: Congressional Budget Office; staff of the Joint Committee on Taxation.

Note: CHIP = Children's Health Insurance Program.

changes in the expected characteristics of plans that will be offered in the exchanges (which will make them less attractive than previously expected).

CBO and JCT project that the government's costs for exchange subsidies and related spending in 2014 will be $3 billion (or 16 percent) less than previously projected. Despite projecting that slightly more people will receive insurance coverage through exchanges over the 2015–2024 period than they had anticipated previously, CBO and JCT project that costs for exchange subsidies and related spending will be $164 billion (or 14 percent) below the previous projection, mainly because of the downward revision to expected exchange premiums, as follows:

■ Premium assistance tax credits total $855 billion in the current projection, a reduction of $181 billion (or 17 percent) from the previous projection.[27]

■ Cost-sharing subsidies are now projected to be $175 billion, about $8 billion more than in the previous projection; that change is attributable to the

slight downward shift in the expected income distribution.

■ The risk corridor program is expected to have no net budgetary effect over the three years of its operation, rather than the $8 billion in net savings to the government previously anticipated.

Medicaid and CHIP Outlays. CBO and JCT's projection of the federal cost of the additional enrollment in Medicaid and CHIP under the ACA has changed little since the February 2014 projection. For 2014, the projection was revised from $19 billion to $20 billion; for the 2015–2024 period, the projection remains at $792 billion. The negligible net revision reflects a combination of offsetting changes in enrollment and per capita costs.

For 2014 through 2016, CBO and JCT have reduced their projections of additional Medicaid and CHIP enrollment stemming from the ACA by about 1 million people each year. For those years, the changes discussed above in the estimated number of people without insurance in the absence of the ACA and the estimated mix of adults and children within that population generated a downward revision in the number of children expected to newly enroll in CHIP and a smaller upward revision in the number of adults expected to newly enroll in Medicaid as a result of the ACA. Because anticipated per capita

---

27. The current estimate is the sum of $726 billion in outlays for the premium credits and a $129 billion reduction in revenues resulting from those credits (see Table 3 on page 10).

costs are much higher for newly eligible adults than for children (and because of some other small technical changes), the projections for federal spending for Medicaid and CHIP have been revised upward by about $2 billion for the 2014–2016 period, despite the downward revision in projected enrollment.

CBO and JCT raised their projections of additional Medicaid enrollment stemming from the ACA by fewer than 1 million people in each year between 2018 and 2024 (for 2017, projected enrollment is essentially unchanged). That revision results mainly from the changes in the projected income distribution and projected labor force participation, discussed above. Higher enrollment would increase federal costs, all else being equal. However, the projection for spending per adult Medicaid recipient has been revised downward slightly on the basis of recent data. The combination of higher enrollment and lower costs per capita led to small upward revisions to projected outlays between 2018 and 2020, to essentially no change in 2021, and to small downward revisions to outlays projected for 2022 through 2024.

Small-Employer Tax Credits. CBO and JCT have made essentially no changes to their projections of small-employer tax credits since February 2014.

Penalty Payments by Uninsured People. Uninsured people are now expected to pay about $6 billion less in penalties during the 2015–2024 period than CBO and JCT projected previously. That reduction is attributable to several factors. First, because of various changes discussed above, the agencies now expect that, in most years, about 1 million fewer people will be uninsured than the agencies expected in February. In addition, a shift in the projected income distribution leaves a smaller share of the uninsured population subject to the penalty, and it leaves fewer people who are subject to the penalty with income high enough that they would pay a percentage of their income as a penalty rather than pay a lesser flat rate. The reduction in projected payments does not result from recent administrative actions to widen the hardship exemption; CBO and JCT expect that those actions will have only negligible effects on payments because most of the people eligible for that exemption will seek alternative sources of coverage rather than become uninsured.

Penalty Payments by Employers. Since preparing the February 2014 projection, CBO and JCT have reduced by $12 billion their estimate of penalty payments that will be collected from employers during the 2015–2024 period. About $3 billion of that reduction occurs in 2016, mainly as a result of the recently issued final rule providing transitional relief for employers (discussed above). The rest is attributable to a small increase in the number of active workers and their dependents who are expected to enroll in employment-based coverage compared with the number in the February baseline.

Excise Tax on High-Premium Insurance Plans. Since February, CBO and JCT have increased by $12 billion their projection of revenues resulting from the excise tax on certain insurance plans with high premiums collected over the 2015–2024 period. That upward revision resulted primarily from an expected increase in the number of active employees receiving employment-based coverage.

Other Effects on Revenues and Outlays. CBO and JCT now anticipate that the ACA's insurance coverage provisions will have other effects on revenues and outlays that will, on net, reduce the deficit by $54 billion less than was anticipated previously for the 2015–2024 period. The current projection is for a reduction in the deficit of $152 billion, rather than $206 billion, for that decade.

The downward revision in those savings stems principally from the projected increase in the number of active workers and their dependents with employment-based health insurance. An employer's decision not to offer insurance to active employees tends to result in higher taxable compensation in the form of wages and salaries. Conversely, an increase in employment-based health insurance tends to reduce taxable compensation. Therefore, the increase in the number of active workers and their dependents with employment-based coverage implies lower federal revenues than would otherwise be the case.

Changes in the Estimates Since the Enactment of the ACA

CBO and JCT have updated their baseline estimates of the budgetary effects of the ACA's insurance coverage provisions many times since that legislation was enacted

Figure 3.

Comparison of CBO and JCT's Estimates of the Net Budgetary Effects of the Coverage Provisions of the Affordable Care Act

(Billions of dollars, by fiscal year)

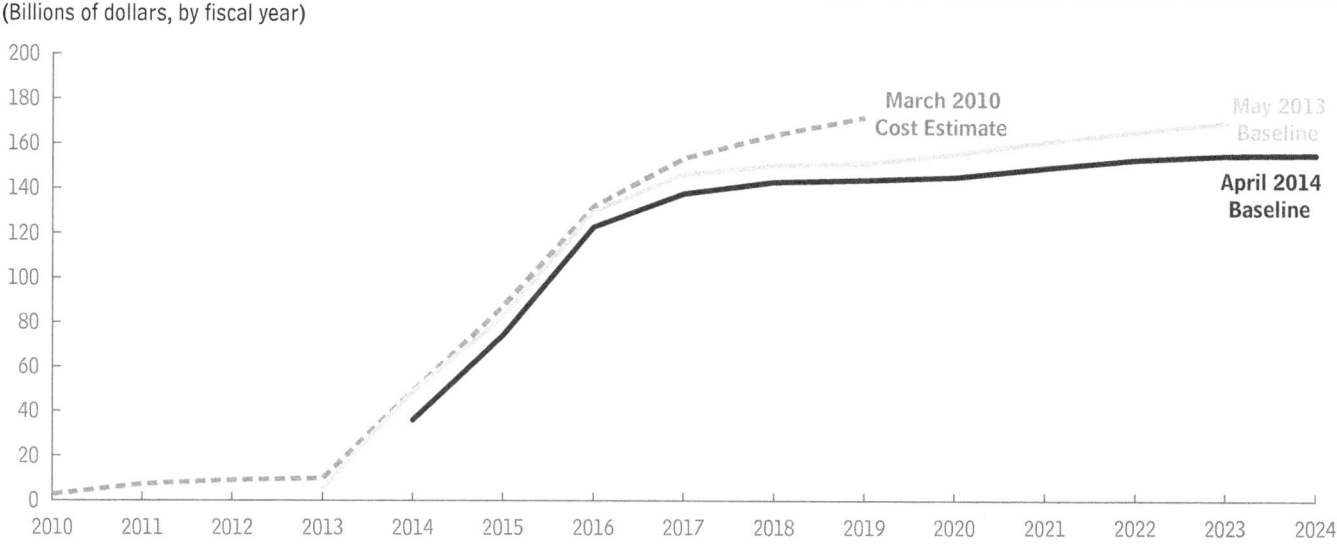

Sources: Congressional Budget Office; staff of the Joint Committee on Taxation.

in March 2010 (see Figure 3). As time has passed, projected costs over the subsequent 10 years have risen because the period spanned by the estimates has changed: Each time a year goes by, a less expensive early year is replaced by a more expensive later year. But when compared year by year, CBO and JCT's estimates of the net budgetary impact of the ACA's insurance coverage provisions have decreased, on balance, over the past four years.[28]

In March 2010, CBO and JCT projected that the provisions of the ACA related to health insurance coverage would cost the federal government $759 billion during fiscal years 2014 through 2019 (2019 was the last year of the 10-year budget window used in that estimate). The newest projections indicate that those provisions will cost $659 billion over that same period, a reduction of

13 percent. For 2019, for example, CBO and JCT projected in March 2010 that the ACA's insurance coverage provisions would have a net federal cost of $172 billion; the current projections show a cost of $144 billion—a reduction of 16 percent.

The net downward revision since March 2010 to CBO and JCT's estimates of the net federal cost of the ACA's insurance coverage provisions (when measured on a year-by-year basis) is attributable to many factors. Changes in law, revisions to CBO's economic projections, judicial decisions, administrative actions, new data, and numerous improvements in CBO and JCT's modeling have all affected the projections. A notable influence is the substantial downward revision to projected health care costs both for the federal government and for the private sector. For example, since early 2010, CBO and JCT have revised downward their projections of insurance premiums for policies purchased through the exchanges in 2016 by roughly 15 percent, and CBO has revised downward its projection of total Medicaid spending per beneficiary in 2016 by roughly half that percentage.

---

28. For an illustration of several baseline projections between March 2010 and May 2013, see Congressional Budget Office, "CBO's Estimate of the Net Budgetary Impact of the Affordable Care Act's Health Insurance Coverage Provisions Has Not Changed Much Over Time," *CBO Blog* (May 14, 2013), www.cbo.gov/publication/44176.

About This Document

This Congressional Budget Office (CBO) report was prepared in response to interest expressed by Members of Congress. In keeping with CBO's mandate to provide objective, impartial analysis, the report makes no recommendations.

Jessica Banthin, Sarah Masi, Eamon Molloy, and Allison Percy prepared the report, with contributions from Kirstin Blom, Stuart Hagen, Jean Hearne, Paul Jacobs, Alexandra Minicozzi, Robert Stewart, Ellen Werble, and the staff of the Joint Committee on Taxation and with guidance from Linda Bilheimer and Peter Fontaine. Philip Ellis and Holly Harvey provided comments.

Robert Sunshine reviewed the report, Kate Kelly edited it, and Maureen Costantino and Jeanine Rees prepared it for publication. The report is available on the agency's website (www.cbo.gov/publication/45231).

Douglas W. Elmendorf
Director

April 2014